POST-PREGNANCY PILATES WORKOUTS GUIDE.

Wall pilates challenge to strengthen & tone your muscles and body plus Exercises to sculpt Abs and glute after pregnancy

Melissa Berry Morre

1

Table Of Contents

INTRODUCTION...**4**

The Benefits Of Post Pregnancy Wall Pilates...........6

Safety Precautions and Guidelines.......................11

CHAPTER ONE... **18**

UNDERSTANDING YOUR POST PREGNANCY BODY...18

CHAPTER TWO..**34**

PREPARING FOR POST-PREGNANCY PILATES 34

CHAPTER THREE.. **50**

Core Strengthening Exercises............................50

CHAPTER FOUR... **69**

Pelvic Floor Exercises.................................... 69

CHAPTER FIVE.. **87**

Importance Of Posture And Alignment.................. 87

CHAPTER SIX... **104**

FULL-BODY STRENGTHENING AND TONING:
Upper Body Exercises with Resistance Bands.....104

Lower Body Exercises for Strength and Stability..110

CHAPTER SEVEN...**124**

FLEXIBILITY AND RELAXATION.........................124

Incorporating Mindfulness into Your Practice....... 136

CHAPTER EIGHT.. **141**

NUTRITION AND HYDRATION TIPS...................141

POST-PREGNANCY PILATES FAQS......................**157**

Common Concerns and Questions Addressed.... 157

MODIFICATIONS FOR SPECIFIC CONDITIONS OR INJURIES.. 164

CELEBRATING YOUR POST-PREGNANCY PILATES JOURNEY.. 170

INTRODUCTION

Welcome and Congratulations!

Congratulations on the birth of your baby and welcome to the wonderful world of post-pregnancy Pilates! This guide is designed to support you on your journey to regain strength, flexibility, and overall well-being after giving birth. By incorporating Pilates into your postpartum routine, you can enhance your physical recovery, improve your posture, and reconnect with your body.

In this guide, we will explore the benefits of post-pregnancy Pilates, provide safety precautions and guidelines, and offer a variety of exercises and techniques specifically tailored to meet the needs of new moms. Whether you are a Pilates enthusiast or new to the practice, this guide will help you navigate the post-pregnancy period and empower you to achieve your fitness goals.

Remember, every woman's postpartum journey is unique, so it's important to listen to your body and progress at your own pace. Take the time to honour and appreciate the incredible journey you've been through, and embrace this opportunity to nurture and care for yourself as you embark on this exciting new chapter.

Let's dive in and discover the transformative power of post-pregnancy Pilates together!

The Benefits Of Post Pregnancy Wall Pilates

The benefits of post-pregnancy Pilates are numerous and can greatly support women in their physical and emotional recovery after giving birth. Here are some key benefits:

1. Restoring Core Strength: Pregnancy and childbirth can weaken the abdominal muscles and lead to diastasis recti (separation of the abdominal muscles). Post-pregnancy Pilates focuses on rebuilding deep core

strength, targeting the transverse abdominis and pelvic floor muscles, which helps improve stability, posture, and overall core strength.

2. Pelvic Floor Rehabilitation: Pilates exercises specifically target the pelvic floor muscles, which can become weakened or damaged during pregnancy and childbirth. By incorporating pelvic floor exercises into your postpartum Pilates routine, you can strengthen and rehabilitate these muscles, improving urinary control and enhancing sexual health.

3. Improving Posture and Alignment: Pregnancy often causes changes in posture and alignment due to the shifting center of gravity and the body's adaptations to accommodate

the growing baby. Post-pregnancy Pilates focuses on alignment, helping to correct postural imbalances, strengthen the back muscles, and improve overall body alignment.

4. Enhancing Flexibility and Range of Motion: Pilates incorporates gentle stretching and lengthening exercises, which can help restore flexibility and improve range of motion in the body. This is particularly beneficial for women who may experience tightness in certain areas, such as the hips, lower back, and shoulders, after childbirth.

5. Promoting Overall Body Strength: Pilates exercises target multiple muscle groups simultaneously, providing a full-body workout. By

engaging in post-pregnancy Pilates, you can regain overall strength and tone your muscles, helping you feel more energized and capable of handling the physical demands of motherhood.

6. Boosting Mood and Reducing Stress: Exercise, including Pilates, has been shown to release endorphins, which can improve mood and reduce stress levels. Post-pregnancy Pilates provides an opportunity for self-care and can contribute to improved mental well-being, helping to alleviate postpartum blues or symptoms of postpartum depression.

7. Restoring Body Confidence: Pregnancy and childbirth can bring about changes in body shape and

self-image. Engaging in post-pregnancy Pilates can help you reconnect with your body, regain strength and control, and foster a positive body image. As you witness the progress and improvements in your physical abilities, you may experience increased body confidence and self-esteem.

It's important to note that every woman's postpartum journey is unique, and it's essential to consult with a healthcare professional or a certified Pilates instructor before starting any exercise program. They can provide guidance specific to your individual needs and ensure that you engage in Pilates safely and effectively.

Safety Precautions and Guidelines

When engaging in post-pregnancy Pilates, it's crucial to prioritise your safety and well-being. Here are some important safety precautions and guidelines to keep in mind:

1. Consult with Your Healthcare Provider: Before starting any exercise program, including post-pregnancy Pilates, it's essential to consult with your healthcare provider. They can assess your individual situation, provide guidance, and ensure that you are physically ready for exercise following childbirth.

2. Start Gradually: Ease into your post-pregnancy Pilates routine

gradually, especially if you're new to Pilates or haven't exercised recently. Begin with gentle exercises and low-impact movements, gradually increasing the intensity and duration over time.

3. Listen to Your Body: Pay attention to your body's signals during exercise. If something feels uncomfortable, painful, or causes any unusual symptoms, stop and seek guidance from a healthcare professional or a certified Pilates instructor. It's important to honor your body's limitations and not push yourself beyond what feels safe and comfortable.

4. Modify and Adapt Exercises: Recognize that your body has gone

through significant changes during pregnancy and childbirth. Modify exercises as necessary to accommodate your postpartum recovery. This may involve using props, such as pillows or blocks, to provide support, or adjusting the range of motion to avoid strain or discomfort.

5. Focus on Core and Pelvic Floor Engagement: Post-pregnancy Pilates places emphasis on rebuilding core strength and pelvic floor health. However, it's crucial to practice proper technique and avoid excessive strain on these areas. Engage the deep core muscles and pelvic floor mindfully, without bearing down or holding your breath. If you have diastasis recti or pelvic floor concerns, consult with a knowledgeable professional who can

guide you through appropriate exercises and modifications.

6. Hydrate and Stay Well-Nourished: Maintain good hydration before, during, and after your Pilates sessions. Drink water regularly to prevent dehydration. Additionally, ensure you're nourishing your body with a well-balanced diet that supports postpartum recovery and provides adequate energy for exercise.

7. Wear Comfortable Clothing: Choose comfortable, breathable clothing that allows for a full range of motion during your Pilates sessions. Supportive sports bras and proper footwear can also contribute to your comfort and safety.

8. Be Mindful of Postpartum Hormones: Postpartum hormones can impact your ligaments and joints, making them more susceptible to injury. Take extra care when stretching or performing movements that involve joint mobility. Avoid overstretching and focus on controlled, gentle movements that respect your body's current capabilities.

9. Seek Professional Guidance: Consider working with a certified Pilates instructor who has experience in post-pregnancy Pilates. They can provide personalized guidance, assess your technique, and offer modifications tailored to your individual needs. Their expertise can help ensure that you're exercising safely and effectively.

Remember, your post-pregnancy Pilates journey is unique, and it's important to prioritise self-care and listen to your body throughout the process. By following these safety precautions and guidelines, you can enjoy the benefits of post-pregnancy Pilates while minimising the risk of injury or discomfort.

CHAPTER ONE

UNDERSTANDING YOUR POST PREGNANCY BODY

During pregnancy, your body undergoes significant hormonal and muscular changes to support the growth and development of your baby. Understanding these changes can help you navigate the post-pregnancy period more effectively. Here are some key hormonal and muscular changes that occur:

1. Hormonal Changes:
   - Progesterone: Progesterone levels rise during pregnancy to support the growth of the uterus and maintain the

pregnancy. It also relaxes smooth muscles, including those in the gastrointestinal tract, leading to slowed digestion and potential constipation.

- Relaxin: Relaxin is a hormone produced by the placenta that increases during pregnancy. It helps relax and loosen the ligaments in the body, particularly around the pelvis, to allow for the baby's passage during childbirth. However, relaxin can also affect other joints and ligaments in the body, making them more vulnerable to strain or injury.

2. Abdominal Muscle Changes:

- Diastasis Recti: Diastasis recti is a condition characterized by the separation of the abdominal muscles, specifically the rectus abdominis, which can occur during pregnancy due to the stretching and expansion of the abdominal wall to accommodate the growing baby. This separation can persist post-pregnancy and may require specific exercises to promote healing and restore abdominal strength.

3. Pelvic Floor Changes:

- Weakening of Pelvic Floor Muscles: The pelvic floor muscles, which support the bladder, uterus, and rectum, can become weakened or stretched during pregnancy and childbirth. This can lead to issues such as urinary incontinence or pelvic organ prolapse.

- Increased Blood Flow: During pregnancy, there is an increased blood flow to the pelvic region, which can contribute to the relaxation and stretching of the pelvic floor muscles.

Understanding these hormonal and muscular changes can help you approach your post-pregnancy exercise routine with caution and focus on exercises that address these specific areas. It's important to consult with a healthcare professional or a certified postnatal exercise specialist, such as a Pilates instructor or physical therapist, who can provide guidance and recommend exercises tailored to your individual needs. By addressing these changes through appropriate exercise and rehabilitation, you can support your body's recovery and regain strength and stability in the post-pregnancy period.

Diastasis Recti: Definition and Management

Diastasis recti is a condition characterized by the separation of the abdominal muscles, specifically the rectus abdominis, which run vertically along the front of the abdomen. It commonly occurs during pregnancy as the growing uterus puts pressure on the abdominal wall, causing the muscles to stretch and separate. Diastasis recti can manifest as a visible gap or bulge between the left and right sides of the abdominal muscles.

Here are some key points regarding the management of diastasis recti:

1. Diagnosis: Diastasis recti can be diagnosed by a healthcare professional

through a physical examination. They will assess the width and depth of the separation and determine the appropriate management approach.

2. Posture and Body Mechanics: Maintaining good posture and practicing proper body mechanics throughout the day can help minimize the strain on the abdominal muscles. Avoid movements and positions that put excessive stress on the midsection, such as heavy lifting or intense abdominal exercises.

3. Core Strengthening Exercises: Engaging in specific exercises that target the deep core muscles can help to strengthen and support the abdominal muscles, including the transverse abdominis. These exercises

should be performed with proper technique and alignment to avoid further separation of the abdominal muscles. Working with a certified postnatal fitness professional or physical therapist who specializes in diastasis recti management can provide guidance on appropriate exercises and modifications.

4. Pelvic Floor Rehabilitation: The pelvic floor muscles and the abdominal muscles work together to provide stability and support to the core. Incorporating pelvic floor exercises, such as Kegels, into your routine can help strengthen these muscles and promote overall core stability.

5. Gradual Progression: It's important to progress gradually when working to heal diastasis recti. Rushing into intense abdominal exercises too soon can potentially worsen the condition. Start with gentle exercises that focus on activating the deep core muscles and gradually increase the intensity and difficulty over time.

6. Supportive Garments: Wearing supportive garments, such as abdominal binders or specialized postnatal compression garments, can provide temporary support to the abdominal muscles and help promote healing. These garments should be used under the guidance of a healthcare professional.

7. Patience and Persistence: Healing diastasis recti takes time and varies for each individual. It's important to be patient with the process and remain consistent with your exercise routine. Results may not be immediate, but with dedication and proper management, improvement is possible.

It's crucial to consult with a healthcare professional or a certified postnatal fitness specialist who can assess your diastasis recti and provide personalized guidance. They can create a tailored exercise program and offer recommendations based on the severity of your condition and your individual needs. By following proper management techniques, you can promote healing and strengthen the abdominal muscles, supporting your overall post-pregnancy recovery.

Pelvic Floor Health and Rehabilitation

Pelvic floor health and rehabilitation are essential aspects of post-pregnancy recovery. The pelvic floor muscles, located at the base of the pelvis, play a crucial role in supporting the pelvic organs, maintaining urinary and bowel control, and enhancing sexual function. Pregnancy and childbirth can weaken the pelvic floor muscles, leading to issues such as urinary incontinence, pelvic organ prolapse, or decreased sensation during intercourse. Here are some key points regarding pelvic floor health and rehabilitation:

1. Pelvic Floor Exercises: Pelvic floor exercises, also known as Kegel exercises, involve contracting and relaxing the muscles of the pelvic floor. These exercises can help strengthen and tone the pelvic floor muscles, improving their function and reducing the risk of pelvic floor disorders. To perform Kegels, identify the muscles used to control urination and try to contract and lift them without engaging the abdominal, buttock, or thigh muscles. Hold the contraction for a few seconds and then release. Gradually increase the duration and number of repetitions over time.

2. Proper Technique: It's crucial to practice proper technique when performing pelvic floor exercises. Focus on isolating the pelvic floor muscles without straining or holding your breath. Avoid squeezing the buttocks, thighs, or abdominal muscles during the exercises. If you're not sure if you're performing the exercises correctly, consider consulting with a healthcare professional or a pelvic floor physical therapist who can provide guidance and feedback.

3. Gradual Progression: Start with gentle pelvic floor exercises and gradually increase the intensity and duration over time. Just like any other muscle group, the pelvic floor muscles need progressive training to build

strength. However, be mindful not to overexert or fatigue the muscles, as this can lead to further issues. Finding the right balance between challenging the muscles and allowing for adequate rest is important.

4. Incorporate Functional Movements: In addition to isolated pelvic floor exercises, it's beneficial to incorporate functional movements into your routine that engage the pelvic floor muscles. Activities such as squats, lunges, and bridges can help strengthen the entire core, including the pelvic floor.

5. Seek Professional Guidance: If you're experiencing significant pelvic floor issues or have concerns about your pelvic floor health, it's advisable

to seek guidance from a healthcare professional or a pelvic floor physical therapist. They can evaluate your pelvic floor function, provide personalized advice, and recommend specific exercises or techniques tailored to your needs.

6. Lifestyle Considerations: Certain lifestyle factors can impact pelvic floor health. Maintaining a healthy weight, avoiding constipation, practicing good posture, and lifting heavy objects properly can all contribute to pelvic floor well-being. Additionally, managing chronic coughing or sneezing, which can put strain on the pelvic floor, is important.

Remember, pelvic floor health and rehabilitation take time and consistency. Be patient and persistent in your efforts, and don't hesitate to seek professional help if needed. Taking care of your pelvic floor can have long-term benefits for your overall well-being and quality of life.

CHAPTER TWO

PREPARING FOR POST-PREGNANCY PILATES

Medical Clearance and Consultation

Before engaging in any post-pregnancy exercise program, including Pilates, it's essential to obtain medical clearance from your healthcare provider. This is particularly important if you had a complicated pregnancy, childbirth, or any medical conditions that may affect your ability to exercise.

Here are some key steps to consider when preparing for post-pregnancy Pilates:

1. Medical Clearance: Schedule a postnatal check-up with your healthcare provider, typically around 6 weeks after childbirth, to ensure that your body has sufficiently healed and that there are no underlying medical concerns that could impact your ability to exercise. Your healthcare provider can assess your overall health, pelvic floor function, and diastasis recti, and provide specific recommendations regarding exercise.

2. Consultation with a Certified Postnatal Pilates Instructor: After receiving medical clearance, it's beneficial to seek guidance from a

certified postnatal Pilates instructor. These professionals have specialized knowledge and training in working with post-pregnancy bodies and can tailor exercises to address specific needs such as diastasis recti, pelvic floor weakness, and overall core strength. They can also provide modifications and progressions based on your individual abilities and goals.

3. Communicate Your Goals and Concerns: During your consultation with a postnatal Pilates instructor, be sure to communicate your goals and any concerns you may have. Whether you're looking to regain core strength, address diastasis recti, or improve pelvic floor function, sharing this information will help the instructor create a personalized program that

aligns with your needs and helps you achieve your desired outcomes.

4. Assessing Diastasis Recti and Pelvic Floor Function: A certified postnatal Pilates instructor will typically assess the severity of diastasis recti and evaluate pelvic floor function. This assessment will help determine the appropriate exercises, modifications, and progression for your specific condition.

5. Start with Gentle Pilates Exercises: In the initial stages of post-pregnancy Pilates, it's important to focus on gentle exercises that gradually reintroduce movements and engage the deep core muscles. The emphasis should be on proper alignment, breathing techniques, and activating

the pelvic floor and deep abdominal muscles.

6. Gradual Progression: As your body becomes stronger and more stable, your postnatal Pilates instructor will guide you through a gradual progression of exercises, increasing the intensity and challenge over time. It's important to listen to your body, take breaks when needed, and avoid pushing yourself beyond your limits.

Remember, every post-pregnancy journey is unique, and it's essential to approach postnatal Pilates with care and guidance from professionals who specialize in postnatal exercise. By obtaining medical clearance, consulting with a certified postnatal Pilates instructor, and gradually progressing your exercise routine, you can safely and effectively regain strength, improve core stability, and support your overall post-pregnancy recovery.

Selecting Appropriate Pilates Equipment and Props

When selecting Pilates equipment and props for your post-pregnancy practice, it's important to consider your individual needs, goals, and any specific recommendations from your healthcare provider or certified postnatal Pilates instructor. Here are some factors to consider when choosing appropriate equipment and props:

1. Mat: A Pilates mat is a fundamental piece of equipment for floor-based exercises. Look for a mat that provides adequate cushioning and support for your body. Consider options with extra thickness or added padding to ensure comfort, especially if you're experiencing any joint or pelvic floor discomfort post-pregnancy.

2. Pilates Reformer: The Pilates reformer is a versatile piece of equipment that uses a sliding carriage, springs, and various attachments to provide resistance and support during exercises. If you have access to a Pilates studio or gym with reformer machines, consult with your postnatal Pilates instructor to determine when it's appropriate to start using the reformer and if any modifications are

needed to accommodate your post-pregnancy needs.

3. Stability Ball: Stability balls, also known as exercise balls or Swiss balls, can be used to challenge balance, stability, and core strength. They can be particularly useful during post-pregnancy Pilates as they engage multiple muscle groups, including the deep core and pelvic floor muscles. Choose a stability ball that is the appropriate size for your height and weight, ensuring that your knees form a 90-degree angle when sitting on the ball.

4. Resistance Bands: Resistance bands provide gentle resistance and can be used to add variety and challenge to your Pilates exercises. They are

lightweight, portable, and come in different levels of resistance. Select bands that offer a suitable level of resistance for your current strength and fitness level, and consider options with handles or loops for ease of use.

5. Small Props: Various small props can be used to add variety and intensify your Pilates workouts. These may include foam rollers, Pilates circles (also known as magic circles or fitness rings), and light hand weights. Consult with your postnatal Pilates instructor to determine when it's appropriate to incorporate these props and how to use them safely and effectively.

6. Props for Pelvic Floor Exercises: For specific pelvic floor exercises, you may

benefit from additional props such as pelvic floor exercise balls or weighted vaginal cones. These props can be used to provide resistance and aid in strengthening the pelvic floor muscles. However, it's important to consult with a pelvic floor specialist or healthcare provider for guidance on using such props safely and effectively.

Remember, when selecting Pilates equipment and props, it's important to prioritize safety, comfort, and appropriateness for your post-pregnancy condition. Consult with your healthcare provider or certified postnatal Pilates instructor for personalized recommendations based on your individual needs, goals, and any specific considerations related to your post-pregnancy recovery.

Creating a Supportive Exercise Environment

Creating a supportive exercise environment is crucial for maintaining motivation, ensuring safety, and enjoying your post-pregnancy workouts. Here are some tips to help you create a supportive exercise environment:

1. Clear and Safe Space: Designate a specific area in your home or find a gym or studio that provides a clean, clutter-free, and safe space for your workouts. Ensure that the area is free from hazards and has enough room for you to move comfortably during your exercises.

2. Proper Lighting and Ventilation: Good lighting is essential for safety and proper form during your workouts. Choose a space with adequate natural or artificial lighting. Additionally, ensure proper ventilation to maintain a comfortable and breathable environment.

3. Supportive Equipment: Invest in exercise equipment and props that are suitable for your post-pregnancy needs and goals. Select items that provide comfort, safety, and appropriate support for your body during workouts. Consider items such as a supportive exercise mat, comfortable workout clothing, and well-fitting athletic shoes.

4. Motivating Music or Audio: Create a playlist of uplifting and energizing music that motivates you during your workouts. Music can help set the mood, boost your energy levels, and make your exercise sessions more enjoyable. Alternatively, you can listen to podcasts, audiobooks, or educational content related to fitness or post-pregnancy wellness to keep you engaged and informed.

5. Time Management: Set aside dedicated time for your workouts and create a schedule that works for you. Prioritize your exercise sessions and treat them as important appointments. This will help you establish a routine and ensure that you have enough time to focus on your well-being.

6. Seek Support: Engage in exercise activities with a workout buddy or join postnatal exercise classes or groups where you can connect with other individuals who are going through a similar post-pregnancy journey. Sharing experiences, challenges, and successes can provide motivation, accountability, and a sense of community.

7. Positive Mindset: Cultivate a positive mindset towards your post-pregnancy exercise journey. Focus on the progress you make, celebrate small victories, and be kind to yourself when facing challenges. Surround yourself with positive affirmations and visual reminders of your goals to help maintain a positive attitude.

8. Professional Guidance: Consider working with a certified postnatal fitness professional, such as a postnatal Pilates instructor or personal trainer, who can provide expert guidance, support, and motivation tailored to your specific needs. They can help you develop a safe and effective exercise program, monitor your progress, and provide feedback to ensure you're on the right track.

By creating a supportive exercise environment, you can enhance your post-pregnancy exercise experience, stay motivated, and enjoy the benefits of physical activity while taking care of your overall well-being.

CHAPTER THREE

Core Strengthening Exercises

Engaging the deep core muscles is essential for effective core strengthening exercises. These muscles include the transverse abdominis, multifidus, pelvic floor muscles, and diaphragm. Here are some techniques to help you engage and activate your deep core muscles:

1. Diaphragmatic Breathing: Start by lying on your back with your knees bent and feet flat on the floor. Place one hand on your chest and the other hand on your abdomen. Take a deep breath in through your nose, allowing your abdomen to rise as you fill your

lungs with air. Exhale slowly through your mouth, gently drawing your navel towards your spine and feeling your abdomen flatten. Focus on breathing deeply into your lower abdomen and feeling the gentle engagement of your deep core muscles.

2. Pelvic Floor Engagement: The pelvic floor muscles are an integral part of your deep core. To engage them, imagine stopping the flow of urine midstream or preventing the passing of gas. You should feel a gentle lifting and squeezing sensation in the pelvic area. It's important not to over-engage or strain the pelvic floor muscles; aim for a gentle contraction.

3. Transverse Abdominis Activation: The transverse abdominis is a deep

abdominal muscle that acts like a corset, providing stability and support to the spine and pelvis. To activate it, imagine gently pulling your belly button in towards your spine without holding your breath or tensing other muscles. Practice this activation while maintaining relaxed breathing.

4.	Multifidus	Activation:	The multifidus muscles are deep back muscles that stabilize the spine. To engage them, imagine lengthening and gently lifting the muscles along the spine. You should feel a subtle sensation of support and lengthening in your lower back.

5. Integrated Core Engagement: Once you have practiced engaging each of the individual deep core muscles,

focus on integrating them together. Start by engaging your pelvic floor, then add the transverse abdominis activation, and finally, incorporate the multifidus engagement. Practice maintaining this integrated core engagement while performing various movements and exercises.

It's important to note that deep core engagement should be a gentle contraction without excessive tension or straining. Avoid holding your breath or creating excessive pressure in the abdomen. Start with shorter holds and gradually increase the duration as you gain strength and control.

Incorporating deep core engagement into your core strengthening exercises, such as Pilates, planks, or stability ball exercises, will enhance their effectiveness and help you develop a strong and stable core. It's recommended to work with a certified postnatal Pilates instructor or a qualified fitness professional who can provide guidance and ensure you're performing the exercises correctly and safely.

Pelvic Tilts and Clocks

Pelvic tilts and pelvic clocks are exercises that can help strengthen and mobilize the pelvic area, improve pelvic stability, and enhance awareness of pelvic alignment. They are particularly beneficial for post-pregnancy recovery and core strengthening. Here's how to perform pelvic tilts and pelvic clocks:

1. Pelvic Tilts:
   - Start by lying on your back with your knees bent and feet flat on the floor, hip-width apart.
   - Relax your body and find a neutral pelvis position, where your natural curves are present and your lower back has a slight arch.
   - Inhale to prepare, and as you exhale, gently tilt your pelvis by flattening your lower back against the floor.
   - Imagine bringing your pubic bone towards your belly button and feel your lower abdominal muscles engage.
   - Hold this position for a moment, maintaining a gentle contraction, and

then inhale to release the tilt and return to the neutral position.

- Repeat this movement for a prescribed number of repetitions or as recommended by your instructor.

2. Pelvic Clocks:

- Begin in the same starting position as the pelvic tilts, lying on your back with knees bent and feet flat on the floor.

- Visualize a clock face on your pelvis, with your belly button as the center point.

- Imagine that you are tracing the numbers on the clock with your pubic bone. Start by tilting your pelvis forward, bringing your pubic bone towards the 12 o'clock position.

- From there, move to the 3 o'clock position by tilting your right hip and bringing your right hip bone towards your right shoulder.

- Continue the movement around the clock, tilting your pelvis back to 6 o'clock, then to 9 o'clock, and finally returning to the 12 o'clock position.

- Reverse the direction and repeat the movement in the opposite direction.

- Focus on maintaining control and stability throughout the movement, engaging the deep core muscles and maintaining relaxed breathing.

Both pelvic tilts and pelvic clocks can be performed as standalone exercises or incorporated into a larger routine. They help improve pelvic mobility, strengthen the deep core muscles, and promote overall pelvic stability. It's important to start with small movements and gradually increase the range of motion as you become more comfortable and gain strength. Always listen to your body and avoid any movements or positions that cause pain or discomfort. If you have any concerns or specific post-pregnancy considerations, consult with a certified postnatal Pilates instructor or healthcare provider for personalized guidance.

Modified Plank Variations

Modified plank variations are excellent for building core strength, stability, and endurance, especially during post-pregnancy recovery. Here are a few modified plank variations that can be more accessible and suitable for individuals with specific needs or who are working on rebuilding core strength:

1. Knee Plank:
   - Start on all fours with your hands directly under your shoulders and knees under your hips.
   - Step your feet back, keeping your knees on the ground. Your body should form a straight line from your head to your knees.
   - Engage your core, draw your shoulder blades down and back, and maintain a neutral spine.
   - Hold this position for a certain duration or as long as you can maintain proper form and breath control.

2. Forearm Plank:

- Begin by kneeling on the floor and place your forearms on the ground, shoulder-width apart.

- Extend your legs behind you, resting on the balls of your feet.

- Engage your core, squeeze your glutes, and maintain a straight line from your head to your heels.

- Keep your elbows directly under your shoulders and avoid sinking or lifting your hips.

- Hold this position for a designated period of time, focusing on maintaining proper alignment and controlled breathing.

3. Elevated Plank:

- Find a sturdy elevated surface, such as a bench, step, or sturdy chair.

- Place your hands on the elevated surface, shoulder-width apart, and step your feet back to a plank position.

- Engage your core, maintain a straight line from your head to your heels, and avoid sagging or lifting your hips.

- Keep your shoulders directly over your wrists and maintain a strong, stable position.

- Hold the elevated plank for a prescribed duration, focusing on maintaining proper form and breathing.

4. Wall Plank:

- Stand facing a wall and place your hands flat against the wall, shoulder-width apart, at shoulder height.

- Step your feet back, keeping your body straight and aligned.
- Engage your core, glutes, and legs, and press your hands firmly against the wall.
- Maintain a straight line from your head to your heels, avoiding any sagging or lifting of the hips.
- Hold the wall plank for a designated period, focusing on maintaining proper alignment and controlled breathing.

Remember, it's important to listen to your body and work within your own comfort and ability level. Start with modifications that feel appropriate for you and gradually progress to more challenging variations as your core strength improves. If you have any concerns or specific post-pregnancy considerations, consult with a certified postnatal Pilates instructor or healthcare provider for personalized guidance and modifications tailored to your needs.

Leg Slides and Scissors

Leg slides and scissors are exercises that target the core, particularly the abdominal muscles, while also engaging the hip flexors and leg muscles. Here's how to perform leg slides and scissors:

1. Leg Slides:
   - Start by lying on your back with your legs extended and your arms by your sides.
   - Engage your core by gently drawing your navel toward your spine.

- Bend one knee and slide your foot along the floor, bringing your knee toward your chest.

- Slowly straighten your leg and slide it back to the starting position, maintaining control and keeping your core engaged.

- Repeat the movement with the opposite leg, alternating between legs for the desired number of repetitions.

2. Scissors:

- Begin by lying on your back with your legs extended and your arms by your sides.

- Engage your core and lift both legs off the floor, keeping them straight and together.

- Lower one leg toward the floor while keeping the other leg lifted.

- Before the lowered leg touches the floor, lift it back up while simultaneously lowering the other leg.
        - Continue alternating the movement, mimicking a scissor-like action with your legs, while maintaining control and engaging your core.
   - Aim to keep your lower back pressed into the floor throughout the exercise.

For both leg slides and scissors, it's important to focus on maintaining proper form and controlled movements. Here are a few additional tips:

- Keep your core engaged throughout the exercises to provide stability and support for your lower back.

- Avoid arching your lower back or allowing it to lift off the floor.

- Breathe naturally and continuously throughout the movements.

- Start with a range of motion that is comfortable for you, gradually increasing it as you build strength and flexibility.

- If you experience any discomfort or strain in your lower back, modify the movement by reducing the range of motion or performing the exercise with bent knees.

As always, it's advisable to consult with a certified postnatal Pilates instructor or healthcare provider to ensure that these exercises are appropriate for your post-pregnancy recovery and to receive personalized

guidance based on your unique needs
and abilities.

CHAPTER FOUR

Pelvic Floor Exercises

Understanding the pelvic floor muscles is crucial for effectively performing pelvic floor exercises. The pelvic floor is a group of muscles that form a hammock-like structure at the base of the pelvis, providing support for the pelvic organs (bladder, uterus, and rectum) and playing a role in urinary and bowel control, sexual function, and stability of the core.

Here are some key points to understand about the pelvic floor muscles:

1. Location: The pelvic floor muscles are located between the pubic bone at the front of the pelvis and the coccyx (tailbone) at the back. They span from side to side, forming a diamond-shaped area.

2. Layers: The pelvic floor muscles consist of three layers: superficial, intermediate, and deep. The deep layer, also known as the levator ani muscles, is the most important for providing support and control.

3. Muscle Types: The pelvic floor muscles contain both fast-twitch and slow-twitch muscle fibers. The slow-twitch fibers provide endurance and support, while the fast-twitch fibers contribute to rapid contractions

during activities like coughing or sneezing.

4. Functions: The pelvic floor muscles have a variety of functions. They help control the release of urine and stool, maintain continence, support the pelvic organs, stabilize the pelvis and spine, and enhance sexual function.

5. Engagement: To engage the pelvic floor muscles, imagine stopping the flow of urine midstream or preventing the passing of gas. You should feel a gentle lifting and squeezing sensation in the pelvic area. It's important to avoid excessive tension or straining of these muscles.

6. Relaxation: Just as important as engaging the pelvic floor muscles is

learning to relax them fully. This is especially important during childbirth and for maintaining healthy muscle tone and function.

7. Training: Pelvic floor exercises, often referred to as Kegel exercises, involve consciously contracting and relaxing the pelvic floor muscles. Regular practice can help strengthen the muscles and improve their control and coordination.

Understanding the anatomy and function of the pelvic floor muscles is crucial for performing pelvic floor exercises correctly and effectively. If you have any concerns or specific pelvic floor issues, it's advisable to consult with a pelvic floor physical therapist or healthcare provider who can provide personalized guidance and ensure you're performing the exercises correctly.

Kegels and Pelvic Floor Contractions

Kegel exercises, also known as pelvic floor exercises, are a series of contractions and relaxations of the pelvic floor muscles. These exercises aim to strengthen and improve the control and coordination of the pelvic floor. Here's how to perform Kegels and pelvic floor contractions:

1. Identify the Pelvic Floor Muscles:

   - Before starting the exercises, it's important to locate the pelvic floor muscles. One way to do this is by attempting to stop the flow of urine midstream. The muscles you engage to do this are the pelvic floor muscles.

2. Find a Comfortable Position:

- You can perform Kegels in various positions, such as sitting, standing, or lying down. Choose a position that is comfortable for you and allows you to focus on the pelvic floor muscles.

3. Perform the Contractions:

- Start by inhaling deeply, then exhale slowly to relax your body.

- Contract the pelvic floor muscles by squeezing and lifting them as if you're trying to stop the flow of urine or prevent the passing of gas.

- Focus on lifting and squeezing the muscles upward, rather than pushing down or tensing the buttocks, thighs, or abdominal muscles.

- Hold the contraction for a few seconds (start with 3-5 seconds), maintaining a steady and controlled effort.

- Release the contraction and fully relax the pelvic floor muscles.

4. Repetitions and Sets:

- Aim to perform 10-15 repetitions of pelvic floor contractions in one session.

- Gradually increase the duration of each contraction over time, aiming for 10 seconds or more.

- Start with one set of exercises per day and gradually work your way up to 3-4 sets throughout the day.

Tips for Effective Kegels and Pelvic Floor Contractions:

- Focus on isolating the pelvic floor muscles and avoid tensing other muscle groups.

- Breathe naturally and avoid holding your breath during the contractions.

- Maintain a relaxed posture throughout the exercises, avoiding unnecessary tension in other parts of your body.

- Consistency is key. Aim to perform Kegels regularly, ideally daily, for optimal results.

- If you're unsure if you're performing Kegels correctly or have specific concerns, consider consulting with a pelvic floor physical therapist or healthcare provider for guidance and personalized instruction.

Remember, Kegels and pelvic floor contractions can be beneficial for both women and men in various stages of life, including during pregnancy, postpartum recovery, and for addressing issues like urinary incontinence or pelvic floor weakness.

Bridge Pose and Pelvic Floor Activation

Bridge pose is a yoga posture that can help activate and strengthen the pelvic floor muscles while also engaging the glutes, hamstrings, and core. Here's how to perform Bridge pose with a focus on pelvic floor activation:

1. Start by lying on your back with your knees bent and feet flat on the floor. Your feet should be hip-width apart,

and your arms should be relaxed by your sides.

2. Engage your core muscles by gently drawing your navel toward your spine. This will help stabilize your pelvis and protect your lower back.

3. Press your feet into the floor, rooting through your heels, and lift your hips off the ground. As you lift, imagine lengthening your tailbone toward your knees to maintain a neutral spine.

4. As you hold the bridge position, focus on activating your pelvic floor muscles. Imagine lifting and drawing them inward, as if you're trying to lift them toward your belly button. This

engages the deep muscles of the pelvic floor.

5. Maintain the bridge position and the engagement of your pelvic floor muscles for a few breaths or as long as you feel comfortable and can maintain proper form.

6. Slowly lower your hips back down to the ground, vertebra by vertebra, with control.

Tips for Bridge Pose and Pelvic Floor Activation:

- Keep your knees aligned with your feet, avoiding them from collapsing inward or splaying outward.

- Avoid excessive tension in your neck, shoulders, and jaw. Keep your upper body relaxed.

- Breathe deeply and naturally throughout the pose, allowing your breath to support the activation of your pelvic floor muscles.

- Start with holding the bridge pose for a few breaths and gradually increase the duration as your strength and comfort level improve.

- If you experience any discomfort or strain in your lower back, modify the pose by lifting your hips to a height that feels comfortable for you.

Bridge pose can be a beneficial exercise for pelvic floor activation and strengthening, but it's important to listen to your body and work within your own comfort and ability level. If you have any specific concerns or conditions related to your pelvic floor, it's advisable to consult with a certified yoga instructor or pelvic floor physical therapist for personalized guidance and modifications tailored to your needs.

Pelvic Floor Release and Relaxation Techniques

Pelvic floor release and relaxation techniques are valuable for promoting relaxation, reducing tension, and improving flexibility in the pelvic floor muscles. Here are some techniques you can try:

1. Deep Breathing:
   - Find a comfortable position, either sitting or lying down.

- Take slow, deep breaths, inhaling deeply through your nose and exhaling through your mouth.

- As you breathe, consciously focus on relaxing your pelvic floor muscles with each exhale.

- Imagine the tension melting away from the pelvic area as you continue to breathe deeply and relax.

2. Pelvic Floor Drops:

- Begin in a seated position with your feet flat on the floor.

- Inhale deeply, and as you exhale, consciously let go of any tension in your pelvic floor.

- Visualize your pelvic floor muscles releasing and dropping downward with each exhale.

- Repeat this exercise several times, allowing your pelvic floor to relax and release with each breath.

3. Pelvic Floor Massage:
    - Find a comfortable and private space where you can lie down.
    - Gently massage the muscles in the pelvic floor area using your fingers or a soft massage ball.
    - Apply gentle pressure and circular motions to release tension and promote relaxation.
    - Experiment with different areas of the pelvic floor, including the perineum (the area between the anus and the genitals) and the muscles around the sit bones.

4. Pelvic Floor Stretching:

   - Start by lying on your back with your knees bent and feet flat on the floor.

   - Slowly bring your knees toward your chest, allowing your pelvic floor to stretch gently.

   - You can support your knees with your hands or wrap your arms around your legs, finding a position that feels comfortable for you.

   - Hold the stretch for a few breaths, allowing your pelvic floor muscles to release and lengthen.

   - Slowly release the stretch and return to the starting position.

5. Relaxing Visualization:

   - Close your eyes and visualize your pelvic floor muscles as soft, warm, and relaxed.

- Imagine a sense of openness and spaciousness in the pelvic area.

- As you continue to visualize, allow any tension or discomfort to dissolve, leaving behind a feeling of deep relaxation and ease.

It's important to note that these techniques may not be suitable for everyone, especially if you have specific pelvic floor conditions or concerns. If you have any pelvic floor-related issues or questions, it's advisable to consult with a pelvic floor physical therapist or healthcare provider who can provide personalized guidance and ensure that these techniques are appropriate for your situation.

CHAPTER FIVE

Importance Of Posture And Alignment

Proper posture and alignment are essential for maintaining optimal musculoskeletal health, preventing injuries, and promoting overall well-being. Here are some key reasons why proper alignment is important:

1. Spinal Health: Proper alignment helps maintain the natural curves of the spine, which are crucial for distributing forces evenly and reducing the risk of strain or injury. Good posture aligns the head, neck, shoulders, and pelvis in a balanced

and neutral position, minimizing stress on the spine.

2. Muscle Balance and Function: Correct alignment promotes balanced muscle development and function. When the body is aligned properly, muscles work together efficiently, reducing the load on certain muscles and preventing overuse or strain. This allows for optimal movement and reduces the risk of muscular imbalances.

3. Joint Health: Proper alignment helps distribute weight and forces evenly across the joints, reducing the risk of excessive stress on specific joints. It also helps maintain joint mobility and stability, preventing joint

deterioration and conditions such as osteoarthritis.

4. Breathing and Organ Function: Good posture and alignment provide adequate space for the lungs to expand fully, allowing for efficient breathing. It also allows organs to be properly positioned, facilitating their optimal function and preventing compression or displacement.

5. Energy Efficiency: Proper alignment allows for efficient movement and optimal energy transfer throughout the body. When the body is aligned, muscles and joints can work together harmoniously, reducing energy waste and fatigue.

6. Confidence and Appearance: Maintaining good posture and alignment can enhance one's physical appearance and project confidence. It creates an impression of poise and self-assurance, while slouching or poor alignment can convey a lack of confidence and may impact how others perceive you.

To improve and maintain proper alignment, consider the following tips:

- Be mindful of your posture throughout the day, whether sitting, standing, or walking.
- Align your ears, shoulders, hips, and ankles in a vertical line when standing or sitting.
- Strengthen your core muscles to support proper alignment.

- Avoid prolonged periods of sitting or standing in one position. Take breaks and vary your posture.
- Use ergonomic furniture and equipment that support good posture, such as an ergonomic chair or an adjustable desk.
- Regularly engage in exercises and activities that promote flexibility, strength, and balance.
- Consider seeking guidance from a physical therapist or a posture specialist who can assess your alignment and provide personalized recommendations.

By prioritizing proper alignment and making conscious efforts to maintain good posture, you can support your overall musculoskeletal health, reduce the risk of injuries, and enhance your physical well-being.

Postural Exercises and Corrections

Postural exercises and corrections can help improve posture, strengthen weak muscles, and promote proper alignment. Here are some exercises and techniques that can aid in correcting postural imbalances:

1. Shoulder Blade Squeezes:
   - Stand or sit with your spine tall and your shoulders relaxed.
   - Squeeze your shoulder blades together, as if you're trying to hold a pencil between them.
   - Hold the squeeze for a few seconds, then release.

- Repeat this exercise for several repetitions to strengthen the muscles that retract and stabilize the shoulder blades.

2. Wall Angels:
  - Stand with your back against a wall, feet hip-width apart, and arms relaxed by your sides.
  - Press your entire back against the wall, maintaining the natural curves of your spine.
  - Raise your arms to shoulder height, bending your elbows to 90 degrees, with your palms facing forward.
  - Slowly slide your arms up the wall, keeping your elbows and wrists in contact with the wall as much as possible.
  - Return to the starting position and repeat for several repetitions, focusing

on maintaining good posture and proper alignment throughout the movement.

3. Chin Tucks:
   - Sit or stand with your spine tall and your shoulders relaxed.
   - Gently retract your chin, bringing it back and down as if you're trying to make a double chin.
   - Hold the position for a few seconds, then release.
   - Repeat this exercise for several repetitions to strengthen the muscles that support proper neck alignment.

4. Core Strengthening:
   - A strong core helps support proper posture and alignment.
   - Engage your core muscles by performing exercises such as planks,

bird dogs, or abdominal bracing exercises.

- Strengthening the abdominal, back, and hip muscles can help stabilize the spine and maintain good posture.

5. Stretching:

- Address tight muscles that contribute to poor posture by incorporating stretching exercises into your routine.

- Focus on stretching the chest, shoulders, neck, hip flexors, and hamstrings.

- Examples include chest stretches, shoulder rolls, neck stretches, kneeling hip flexor stretches, and hamstring stretches.

6. Postural Awareness:
 - Throughout the day, be mindful of your posture and make adjustments as needed.
 - Imagine a string pulling you upward from the top of your head, elongating your spine.
 - Avoid slouching or hunching forward, and consciously maintain a neutral spine and aligned posture.

Remember, consistency is key when it comes to postural corrections. Regular practice of these exercises and conscious awareness of your posture can help improve alignment and strengthen the muscles necessary to maintain proper posture. If you have specific postural concerns or conditions, it can be helpful to consult with a physical therapist or posture specialist who can provide personalized guidance and recommendations.

Stretching and Mobilization Techniques

Stretching and mobilization techniques can help improve flexibility, release muscle tension, and promote joint mobility. Here are some effective techniques you can incorporate into your routine:

1. Static Stretching:
   - Static stretching involves holding a stretch for a prolonged period, typically 15-30 seconds, without any bouncing or jerking movements.
   - Focus on stretching the major muscle groups, including the

hamstrings, quadriceps, calves, chest, shoulders, and back.

- Hold each stretch at a point of mild tension, feeling a gentle pull without pain.

- Breathe deeply and relax into the stretch, allowing the muscles to gradually lengthen.

2. Dynamic Stretching:

- Dynamic stretching involves moving through a range of motion in a controlled manner.

- Perform dynamic stretches before a workout or physical activity to warm up the muscles and prepare them for movement.

- Examples include arm circles, walking lunges, leg swings, and torso twists.

- Move smoothly and gradually, avoiding any abrupt or jerky movements.

3. PNF Stretching:

- Proprioceptive Neuromuscular Facilitation (PNF) stretching combines static stretching with muscle contraction and relaxation techniques.

- Start by stretching a muscle group with a static stretch.

- Then, contract the muscles being stretched for about 5-10 seconds, using about 30% of your maximum effort.

- After the contraction, relax the muscles and move deeper into the stretch.

- Repeat this process a few times, gradually increasing the stretch with each repetition.

4. Foam Rolling:

- Foam rolling, also known as self-myofascial release, helps release muscle tension and improve tissue flexibility.

- Using a foam roller, apply pressure to specific areas of your body, such as the calves, quadriceps, hamstrings, and back.

- Roll slowly over the targeted muscle, pausing on any tender or tight spots.

- Apply gentle pressure and avoid rolling over bony areas or joints.

- Perform foam rolling regularly, especially before or after workouts, to promote muscle recovery and flexibility.

5. Joint Mobilization:
    - Joint mobilization techniques involve gentle movements and stretches to improve joint mobility and reduce stiffness.
    - Examples include wrist circles, shoulder rolls, ankle rotations, and spinal twists.
   - Move within your pain-free range of motion, avoiding any forceful or excessive movements.
    - Focus on fluid and controlled motions that gradually increase joint mobility.

6. Yoga and Pilates:
    - Yoga and Pilates incorporate a variety of stretching and mobilization exercises that promote flexibility, strength, and body awareness.

- These practices often involve flowing movements, deep stretches, and controlled breathing techniques.

- Attend yoga or Pilates classes, or follow online tutorials or videos to learn and practice specific poses and sequences.

Remember to listen to your body and stretch within your comfort level. Avoid bouncing or forcing a stretch, as it can lead to injury. If you have any specific concerns or conditions, it's advisable to consult with a healthcare professional or a certified fitness instructor who can provide guidance and modifications tailored to your needs.

CHAPTER SIX

FULL-BODY STRENGTHENING AND TONING: Upper Body Exercises with Resistance Bands

Resistance bands are versatile and effective tools for full-body strengthening and toning, including the upper body. They provide resistance throughout the entire range of motion, helping to build strength, improve muscle tone, and increase overall fitness. Here are some upper body exercises you can perform using resistance bands:

1. Banded Rows:

- Anchor the resistance band securely around a stable object at waist height.

- Stand facing the anchor point, holding the band in both hands with your palms facing each other.

- Step back to create tension in the band, keeping your feet shoulder-width apart.

- Keep your back straight, engage your core, and pull the band towards your body, squeezing your shoulder blades together.

- Slowly release and repeat for a desired number of repetitions.

2. Banded Chest Press:

- Attach the resistance band to a secure anchor point behind you, such as a door handle.

- Stand facing away from the anchor point, holding the band in both hands at chest level.

- Step forward to create tension in the band, keeping your feet hip-width apart.

- Push the band forward, extending your arms fully in front of you.

- Slowly return to the starting position and repeat for a desired number of repetitions.

3. Banded Shoulder Press:

- Stand on the center of the resistance band, holding the ends at shoulder height with your palms facing forward.

- Start with your elbows bent at 90 degrees and your upper arms parallel to the floor.

- Press the band overhead, fully extending your arms.

- Slowly lower the band back to the starting position and repeat for a desired number of repetitions.

4. Banded Bicep Curls:

- Stand on the center of the resistance band, holding the ends with your palms facing forward and your arms fully extended.

- Keeping your upper arms stationary, bend your elbows and curl the band towards your shoulders.

- Slowly lower the band back to the starting position and repeat for a desired number of repetitions.

5. Banded Tricep Pushdowns:

- Attach the resistance band to a secure anchor point above your head.

- Stand facing the anchor point, holding the band in both hands with your palms facing down.

- Start with your elbows bent at 90 degrees and your upper arms close to your body.

- Push the band downward, fully extending your arms.

- Slowly return to the starting position and repeat for a desired number of repetitions.

6. Banded Lateral Raises:

- Stand on the center of the resistance band, holding the ends with your palms facing inward and your arms by your sides.

- Keeping a slight bend in your elbows, raise your arms out to the sides until they are parallel to the floor.

- Slowly lower the band back to the starting position and repeat for a desired number of repetitions.

Remember to start with a resistance band that provides an appropriate level of challenge but still allows you to maintain proper form. As you progress, you can increase the resistance by using a thicker band or adjusting the tension. Perform these exercises in a controlled manner, focusing on quality of movement rather than speed. Additionally, always consult with a healthcare professional or certified fitness instructor before starting any new exercise program, especially if you have any pre-existing conditions or injuries.

Lower Body Exercises for Strength and Stability

Strengthening and stabilizing the lower body is crucial for overall functional fitness and daily activities. Here are some effective lower body exercises that can help improve strength and stability:

1. Squats:
	- Stand with your feet shoulder-width apart, toes slightly turned out.
	- Engage your core, keep your chest lifted, and lower your hips down and back as if sitting into a chair.
	- Keep your knees aligned with your toes and your weight in your heels.

- Lower yourself as far as you can while maintaining good form, then push through your heels to return to the starting position.

- Repeat for a desired number of repetitions.

2. Lunges:

- Start by standing with your feet shoulder-width apart.

- Take a step forward with one foot, ensuring that your knee is directly above your ankle and your front thigh is parallel to the ground.

- Lower your back knee down toward the ground, maintaining an upright torso.

- Push through your front heel to return to the starting position.

- Repeat on the opposite side, alternating legs for a desired number of repetitions.

3. Deadlifts:
- Stand with your feet hip-width apart, holding a barbell or dumbbells in front of your thighs.
- Hinge forward at the hips while maintaining a neutral spine, lowering the weight down toward the ground, keeping it close to your body.
- Engage your glutes and hamstrings to lift your torso back up to a standing position.
- Be mindful of keeping your back straight and your core engaged throughout the movement.
- Repeat for a desired number of repetitions.

4. Step-ups:
  - Stand facing a sturdy step or bench.
  - Step one foot onto the step, driving through your heel and lifting your body up onto the step.
  - Keep your chest lifted and your core engaged.
  - Step back down with the same foot and repeat the movement on the opposite side.
  - Alternate legs for a desired number of repetitions.

5. Glute Bridge:
  - Lie on your back with your knees bent and feet flat on the floor, hip-width apart.
  - Engage your core, squeeze your glutes, and lift your hips off the ground until your body forms a straight line from your knees to your shoulders.

- Pause at the top for a moment, then lower your hips back down to the starting position.

- Repeat for a desired number of repetitions.

6. Calf Raises:

- Stand with your feet hip-width apart, holding onto a stable surface for support if needed.

- Rise up onto the balls of your feet, lifting your heels as high as possible.

- Pause at the top for a moment, then lower your heels back down to the ground.

- Repeat for a desired number of repetitions.

Remember to use proper form and technique for each exercise. Start with a weight or resistance level that challenges you but allows you to maintain good form throughout the movement. Gradually increase the intensity or resistance as your strength improves. If you have any pre-existing conditions or injuries, it's advisable to consult with a healthcare professional or certified fitness instructor before starting a new exercise program.

Total Body Workout Routines

Total body workout routines are an excellent way to target multiple muscle groups, build strength, and improve overall fitness. Here's an example of a total body workout routine that incorporates various exercises:

Note: Before starting any new exercise program, it's important to consult with a healthcare professional or certified fitness instructor, especially if you have any pre-existing conditions or injuries.

Warm-up:
- Begin with 5-10 minutes of light cardio, such as jogging, cycling, or jumping jacks, to increase your heart rate and warm up your muscles.
- Follow the cardio warm-up with dynamic stretches, such as arm circles, leg swings, and torso twists, to further prepare your body for the workout.

1. Squats:
- Stand with your feet shoulder-width apart, toes slightly turned out.
- Engage your core, keep your chest lifted, and lower your hips down and back as if sitting into a chair.

- Keep your knees aligned with your toes and your weight in your heels.
- Lower yourself as far as you can while maintaining good form, then push through your heels to return to the starting position.
- Perform 3 sets of 10-12 repetitions.

2. Push-ups:
- Start in a high plank position with your hands slightly wider than shoulder-width apart, fingers pointing forward.
- Keep your body in a straight line from head to heels, engage your core, and lower your chest toward the ground by bending your elbows.
- Push back up to the starting position, fully extending your arms.

- Modify the exercise by performing push-ups on your knees or against a wall if needed.
- Perform 3 sets of 8-10 repetitions.

3. Bent-Over Rows:
- Hold a dumbbell or kettlebell in each hand, hinge forward at the hips, and maintain a flat back.
- Let your arms hang straight down toward the ground with your palms facing each other.
- Squeeze your shoulder blades together as you pull the weights up toward your chest, keeping your elbows close to your body.
- Lower the weights back down with control.
- Perform 3 sets of 10-12 repetitions.

4. Lunges with Overhead Press:
- Hold a dumbbell or kettlebell in each hand at shoulder height.
- Take a step forward with your right foot and lower into a lunge, keeping your front knee aligned with your ankle.
- As you push back up to the starting position, press the weights overhead, fully extending your arms.
- Repeat the lunge and overhead press on the opposite side.
- Perform 3 sets of 8-10 repetitions on each leg.

5. Plank:
- Start in a high plank position with your hands directly under your shoulders and your body in a straight line.

- Engage your core, squeeze your glutes, and hold the position while maintaining proper form.
- Aim to hold the plank for 30-60 seconds, gradually increasing the duration as you get stronger.
- Perform 3 sets, resting for 30-60 seconds between sets.

6. Russian Twists:
- Sit on the ground with your knees bent and your feet flat on the floor.
- Lean back slightly, engage your core, and lift your feet a few inches off the ground.
- Hold a weight or medicine ball in front of you with both hands.
- Twist your torso to the right, bringing the weight or ball beside your right hip.

- Return to the center and twist to the left, bringing the weight or ball beside your left hip.
- Continue alternating sides for a total of 10-12 repetitions on each side.
- Perform 3 sets.

Cool-down:
- Finish the workout with 5-10 minutes of light cardio, such as walking or stretching exercises, to gradually lower your heart rate and help your muscles recover.

Remember to choose weights or resistance levels that challenge you but allow you to maintain proper form throughout each exercise. Focus on performing each movement with control and precision. As you progress, you can increase the weight or resistance and adjust the number of sets and repetitions to continue challenging your body.

CHAPTER SEVEN

FLEXIBILITY AND RELAXATION

Gentle Stretching for Tight Muscles

After giving birth, gentle stretching can be beneficial for postpartum recovery, promoting flexibility, relaxation, and relieving muscle tightness. Here are some gentle stretching exercises that target commonly tight muscles postpartum:

1. Chest Stretch:
- Stand tall and interlace your fingers behind your back.

- Gently squeeze your shoulder blades together as you lift your arms away from your body.
- Feel the stretch in your chest and shoulders.
- Hold the stretch for 20-30 seconds, breathing deeply.
- Repeat 2-3 times.

2. Seated Forward Fold:
- Sit on the floor with your legs extended in front of you.
- Slowly hinge forward at your hips, reaching towards your toes.
- Allow your head and neck to relax.
- Feel the stretch in your hamstrings and lower back.
- Hold the stretch for 20-30 seconds, breathing deeply.
- Repeat 2-3 times.

3. Child's Pose:
- Start on your hands and knees, with your knees wider than hip-width apart.
- Sit your hips back towards your heels and extend your arms forward, resting your forehead on the mat.
- Relax your entire body and breathe deeply.
- Feel the stretch in your hips, lower back, and shoulders.
- Hold the stretch for 20-30 seconds, breathing deeply.
- Repeat 2-3 times.

4. Hip Flexor Stretch:
- Kneel on one knee, with your other foot flat on the floor in front of you.
- Engage your core and gently push your hips forward, feeling the stretch in the front of your hip and thigh.

- Keep your torso upright and avoid arching your lower back.
- Hold the stretch for 20-30 seconds on each side, breathing deeply.
- Repeat 2-3 times on each side.

5. Cat-Cow Stretch:
- Start on your hands and knees, with your hands directly under your shoulders and your knees under your hips.
- Inhale and arch your back, lifting your chest and tailbone towards the ceiling while dropping your belly towards the floor (Cow Pose).
- Exhale and round your back, tucking your chin towards your chest and drawing your belly button towards your spine (Cat Pose).

- Move slowly and smoothly between Cat and Cow poses, coordinating your breath with the movement.
- Repeat 8-10 times, focusing on the gentle stretch through your spine.

6. Neck and Shoulder Rolls:
- Sit or stand tall with your shoulders relaxed.
- Slowly roll your shoulders forward, up, and back in a circular motion.
- After a few repetitions, reverse the direction and roll your shoulders backward, up, and forward.
- Perform 8-10 rolls in each direction, focusing on releasing tension in your neck and shoulders.

Remember to listen to your body and only stretch to a comfortable level. Avoid any movements or positions that cause pain or discomfort. As a new mother, it's important to start slowly and gradually increase the intensity and duration of your stretching routine as your body heals and regains strength. If you have any concerns or specific postpartum conditions, consult with your healthcare provider before starting any new exercise or stretching program.

Relaxation Techniques and Breathing Exercises

Relaxation techniques and breathing exercises can be highly beneficial for reducing stress, promoting relaxation, and restoring a sense of calm. Here are a few techniques you can try:

1. Deep Breathing:

- Find a comfortable seated position or lie down.

- Close your eyes and take a deep breath in through your nose, filling your belly with air.

- Slowly exhale through your mouth, letting go of any tension or stress.

- Continue breathing deeply and slowly, focusing on the sensation of your breath entering and leaving your body.

- Practice deep breathing for a few minutes or as long as you like, allowing yourself to relax and unwind.

2. Progressive Muscle Relaxation:

- Find a quiet and comfortable space to sit or lie down.

- Starting from your toes, progressively tense and then relax each muscle group in your body.

- Begin by tensing your toes, holding for a few seconds, and then releasing the tension as you exhale slowly.

- Move your focus to your feet, calves, thighs, abdomen, arms, shoulders, and so on, repeating the process of tensing and relaxing each muscle group.

- As you release tension, imagine the stress melting away and a sense of deep relaxation spreading throughout your body.

- Spend a few minutes on this exercise, allowing your body to completely relax.

3. Guided Imagery:

 - Find a quiet and comfortable space where you won't be disturbed.

 - Close your eyes and take a few deep breaths to relax.

 - Imagine yourself in a peaceful and serene setting, such as a beach, forest, or any place that brings you a sense of calm.

 - Engage your senses by visualizing the surroundings, feeling the warmth of the sun, the gentle breeze, or the texture of the ground beneath you.

 - Stay in this imaginary place for a few minutes, allowing yourself to fully immerse in the experience and let go of any stress or worries.

4. Mindfulness Meditation:

 - Find a quiet and comfortable space to sit or lie down.

- Close your eyes and bring your attention to the present moment.

- Focus on your breath, observing each inhalation and exhalation without judgment.

- If your mind wanders, gently bring your attention back to your breath.

- Expand your awareness to the sensations in your body, the sounds around you, and the thoughts passing through your mind.

- Practice mindfulness meditation for a few minutes or longer, allowing yourself to be fully present and accepting of the present moment.

5. Yoga or Stretching:

- Engaging in gentle yoga or stretching exercises can help release tension and promote relaxation.

- Follow a guided yoga routine or perform simple stretches that target areas of your body where you hold tension, such as the neck, shoulders, and hips.

- Focus on slow, deliberate movements, and combine them with deep breathing to enhance the relaxation benefits.

Remember that relaxation techniques and breathing exercises are personal practices, and it may take some experimentation to find the techniques that work best for you. Make time for regular relaxation practice, even if it's just a few minutes each day, to help manage stress and promote overall well-being.

Incorporating Mindfulness into Your Practice

Incorporating mindfulness into your daily life and various activities can help you cultivate a greater sense of presence, awareness, and overall well-being. Here are some ways to incorporate mindfulness into your practice:

1. Mindful Breathing: Take moments throughout the day to bring your attention to your breath. Whether you're sitting, walking, or engaged in any activity, observe the sensation of your breath entering and leaving your body. Focus on the present moment and let go of any distractions or racing thoughts.

2. Mindful Eating: Pay attention to the experience of eating by engaging your senses. Notice the colors, textures, and flavors of your food. Chew slowly and savor each bite, fully experiencing the nourishment it provides. Be present and mindful of your body's hunger and fullness cues.

3. Mindful Movement: Whether you're practicing yoga, going for a walk, or engaging in any physical activity, bring mindfulness to your movements. Notice the sensations in your body, the rhythm of your breath, and the connection between your body and the environment. Stay present and fully engage in the experience.

4. Mindful Work: Bring mindfulness to your work by focusing on one task at a

time. Avoid multitasking and instead give your full attention to each activity. Notice the details, fully engage in the process, and let go of any judgments or distractions.

5. Mindful Communication: Practice mindful communication by truly listening to others without interrupting or preparing your response. Give your full attention to the person speaking, observe their body language, and respond with kindness and compassion. Notice your own thoughts and emotions during conversations without getting carried away by them.

6. Mindful Self-Care: Incorporate mindfulness into your self-care routines. Whether it's taking a bath,

practicing meditation, or engaging in a hobby, be fully present and attentive to the experience. Notice the sensations, emotions, and thoughts that arise, and approach yourself with kindness and self-compassion.

7. Mindful Reflection: Take time each day to reflect on your experiences, thoughts, and emotions. Sit quietly and observe without judgment. Notice any patterns or habits that arise and bring curiosity to your inner landscape. This practice of self-reflection can help you cultivate self-awareness and make conscious choices in your life.

Remember that mindfulness is a skill that develops over time with practice. Start with small moments of mindfulness throughout your day and gradually expand the practice. Be patient and kind to yourself as you cultivate mindfulness, and remember that each moment is an opportunity to be present and engaged in your life.

CHAPTER EIGHT

NUTRITION AND HYDRATION TIPS

Nutritional Requirements for Post-Pregnancy Recovery

Proper nutrition is essential for post-pregnancy recovery as it supports healing, provides energy, and helps replenish nutrient stores. Here are some important nutritional requirements to consider during the postpartum period:

1. Adequate Caloric Intake: While caloric needs vary depending on factors like breastfeeding, activity level, and individual metabolism, it's important to consume enough calories

to support your body's recovery and energy needs. Aim for a balanced and varied diet that includes nutrient-dense foods.

2. Macronutrients:

- Protein: Include adequate protein in your diet to support tissue repair and recovery. Good sources include lean meats, fish, poultry, eggs, dairy products, legumes, nuts, and seeds.

- Carbohydrates: Choose complex carbohydrates like whole grains, fruits, vegetables, and legumes, which provide sustained energy and essential nutrients.

- Healthy Fats: Include sources of healthy fats such as avocados, nuts, seeds, olive oil, and fatty fish, which provide essential fatty acids and support hormone production.

3. Hydration: Stay well-hydrated by drinking plenty of fluids, especially if you are breastfeeding. Aim for water as your primary beverage and limit or avoid sugary drinks. Remember that thirst can sometimes be mistaken for hunger, so ensure you're drinking enough water throughout the day.

4. Essential Nutrients:

- Iron: Iron levels may be depleted after childbirth, especially if there was significant blood loss. Consume iron-rich foods such as lean meats, dark leafy greens, legumes, and fortified cereals to support red blood cell production.

- Calcium: Calcium is important for bone health and breastfeeding mothers. Include dairy products, fortified plant-based milk, leafy greens, and calcium-rich foods in your diet.

- Omega-3 Fatty Acids: Omega-3 fatty acids are beneficial for brain health and may help reduce postpartum mood disorders. Include fatty fish (such as salmon and sardines), walnuts, flaxseeds, and chia seeds in your diet.

- Vitamins and Minerals: Consume a variety of fruits, vegetables, whole grains, and lean proteins to ensure you're getting a broad range of essential vitamins and minerals.

5. Fiber: Include fiber-rich foods like whole grains, fruits, vegetables, legumes, and nuts to support digestion and prevent constipation, which is common postpartum.

It's important to consult with a healthcare professional or a registered dietitian for personalized advice, especially if you have specific dietary needs, medical conditions, or are breastfeeding. They can help tailor your nutrition plan to meet your individual requirements and ensure you are getting the necessary nutrients for optimal post-pregnancy recovery.

Healthy Eating Habits and Meal Planning

Developing healthy eating habits and engaging in meal planning can contribute to overall well-being and make it easier to maintain a nutritious diet. Here are some tips for healthy eating habits and meal planning:

1. Eat a Balanced Diet: Include a variety of nutrient-dense foods from all food groups in your meals. Aim for a balance of carbohydrates, proteins, and healthy fats, along with plenty of fruits and vegetables. This ensures you get a wide range of essential nutrients.

2. Portion Control: Pay attention to portion sizes to avoid overeating. Use smaller plates and bowls, and listen to your body's hunger and fullness cues. Eat until you feel satisfied, not overly stuffed.

3. Focus on Whole Foods: Choose whole foods over processed foods whenever possible. Whole foods are generally less processed and contain more nutrients. Incorporate whole

grains, lean proteins, fresh fruits and vegetables, and healthy fats into your meals.

4. Limit Added Sugars and Sodium: Be mindful of added sugars and sodium in your diet. Read food labels and choose options with lower amounts of added sugars and sodium. Opt for natural sweeteners like fruits and limit your intake of sugary drinks and processed snacks.

5. Cook at Home: Cooking at home gives you control over the ingredients and cooking methods. It allows you to choose healthier options and avoid excessive amounts of unhealthy additives and preservatives. Experiment with new recipes and try

to prepare meals in advance to save time during busy days.

6. Plan Your Meals: Set aside time each week to plan your meals. Consider your schedule, dietary preferences, and nutritional needs. Plan balanced meals that include a variety of ingredients. Make a shopping list based on your meal plan to ensure you have all the necessary ingredients on hand.

7. Batch Cooking and Meal Prep: Consider batch cooking and meal prep to save time and make healthy eating more convenient. Cook larger quantities of meals and portion them out for future meals. Pre-cut vegetables, prepare snacks, and have

healthy options readily available for busy days.

8. Mindful Eating: Practice mindful eating by being present and fully engaged in your meals. Slow down, savor each bite, and pay attention to the flavors, textures, and sensations. Avoid distractions, such as screens or work, and focus on nourishing your body and enjoying the eating experience.

9. Stay Hydrated: Drink plenty of water throughout the day to stay hydrated. Limit sugary drinks and opt for water as your primary beverage. Carry a water bottle with you to ensure you have access to water wherever you go.

10. Seek Professional Advice: If you have specific dietary needs, health concerns, or are unsure how to plan nutritious meals, consult with a registered dietitian. They can provide personalized guidance and help you create a meal plan that suits your needs and goals.

Remember that healthy eating is a long-term commitment and should be approached with a balanced and sustainable mindset. Gradual changes and consistency are key to developing healthy eating habits that are enjoyable and sustainable over time.

Importance of Hydration for Postpartum Exercise and Recovery

Hydration is crucial for postpartum exercise and recovery as it supports various physiological functions and helps optimize overall well-being. Here are some reasons why hydration is important during this period:

1. Replenishes Fluid Loss: The body loses fluids through sweat and increased urine production during exercise. Proper hydration helps replenish these lost fluids and maintain the body's fluid balance.

2. Supports Recovery: Adequate hydration is essential for the body's recovery process after pregnancy and

childbirth. It helps transport nutrients to cells, aids in the removal of waste products, and supports tissue repair and healing.

3. Promotes Milk Production: If you are breastfeeding, staying well-hydrated is important for milk production. Dehydration can affect milk supply, so it's crucial to drink enough fluids to support both your own hydration and the production of breast milk.

4. Regulates Body Temperature: During exercise, the body's temperature rises as a result of increased metabolic activity. Proper hydration helps regulate body temperature and prevents overheating,

which is particularly important during postpartum exercise.

5. Supports Energy Levels: Dehydration can lead to feelings of fatigue and decreased energy levels. By maintaining proper hydration, you can help optimize your energy levels, which is important for daily activities, exercise, and caring for your baby.

6. Promotes Bowel Regularity: Hydration plays a key role in maintaining healthy digestion and preventing constipation, which is a common issue during the postpartum period. Drinking enough fluids can help soften stools and promote regular bowel movements.

7. Enhances Exercise Performance: Being adequately hydrated can improve exercise performance and prevent the negative effects of dehydration, such as reduced endurance, muscle cramps, and fatigue. This can help you engage in postpartum exercise more comfortably and effectively.

Tips for Staying Hydrated:

- Drink water regularly throughout the day, even when you're not exercising.
- Carry a water bottle with you to ensure easy access to fluids.
- Listen to your body's thirst cues and drink when you feel thirsty.
- Consume hydrating foods such as fruits and vegetables, which have high water content.

- Limit or avoid excessive caffeine and alcohol consumption, as these can contribute to dehydration.
- If you're engaging in intense or prolonged exercise, consider a sports drink that contains electrolytes to help replenish lost minerals.

Remember that individual hydration needs can vary, so it's important to listen to your body and adjust your fluid intake accordingly. If you have specific concerns or questions about hydration and exercise during the postpartum period, it's always a good idea to consult with your healthcare provider for personalized guidance.

POST-PREGNANCY PILATES FAQS

Common Concerns and Questions Addressed

Here are some common concerns and questions related to post-pregnancy Pilates, along with their answers:

1. Is it safe to do Pilates after giving birth?

Yes, Pilates can be safe and beneficial after giving birth. However, it's important to wait until your healthcare provider gives you the green light to resume exercise. Generally, it's recommended to wait until at least six weeks postpartum, or longer if you had a complicated delivery or medical concerns.

2. What are the benefits of post-pregnancy Pilates?

Post-pregnancy Pilates can offer several benefits, including:
- Restoring core strength and stability
- Toning and strengthening the pelvic floor muscles
- Improving posture and alignment
- Enhancing overall strength and flexibility
- Aiding in recovery from pregnancy and childbirth
- Promoting relaxation and stress relief

3. Can I start Pilates if I had a C-section?

Yes, Pilates can be started after a C-section, but it's important to follow your healthcare provider's guidance and wait until you have healed sufficiently. You may need to modify certain exercises and avoid putting direct pressure on the incision site during the initial stages of recovery.

4. What type of Pilates is best for post-pregnancy?

Post-pregnancy, it's generally recommended to start with gentle or modified Pilates exercises that focus on core stability, pelvic floor strengthening, and gentle stretching. Mat-based Pilates and specialized postnatal Pilates classes are often suitable options. As you regain strength and stability, you can progress to more challenging exercises with the guidance of a qualified instructor.

5. How soon can I start strengthening my abdominal muscles?

It's important to allow the abdominal muscles time to heal and regain their strength after pregnancy and childbirth. Generally, it's advisable to start with gentle abdominal activation exercises and gradually progress as advised by your healthcare provider or a qualified Pilates instructor. Avoid exercises that cause pain or discomfort.

6. Can Pilates help with diastasis recti?

Yes, Pilates can be effective in addressing diastasis recti, which is the separation of the abdominal muscles that can occur during pregnancy. A qualified instructor can guide you through specific exercises that target the deep core muscles and help promote proper alignment and healing of the abdominal muscles.

7. How frequently should I do post-pregnancy Pilates?

The frequency of your Pilates practice will depend on various factors, including your overall fitness level, recovery progress, and time availability. Initially, starting with 1-2 sessions per week and gradually increasing frequency as you feel comfortable and stronger is a good approach. Listen to your body and allow for adequate rest and recovery.

8. Can Pilates help with postpartum weight loss?

While Pilates can contribute to overall fitness and toning, it's important to note that weight loss primarily depends on a combination of factors, including a balanced diet and regular cardiovascular exercise. Pilates can complement these efforts by improving strength, posture, and body composition.

Remember to consult with your healthcare provider before starting any exercise program, including post-pregnancy Pilates. Additionally, working with a qualified Pilates instructor who has experience with postnatal clients can provide personalized guidance and ensure you're performing exercises safely and effectively.

MODIFICATIONS FOR SPECIFIC CONDITIONS OR INJURIES

When practicing Pilates, modifications may be necessary to accommodate specific conditions or injuries. Here are some common conditions and injuries along with suggested modifications:

1. Pregnancy:

   - Avoid exercises that involve lying flat on your back after the first trimester. Instead, use a wedge or props to elevate your upper body.

   - Modify exercises that put pressure on the abdomen, such as deep twists or intense abdominal work.

- Focus on maintaining good posture, strengthening the pelvic floor, and gentle stretching.

2. Diastasis Recti (Abdominal Separation):
 - Avoid exercises that cause the abdomen to bulge or increase intra-abdominal pressure, such as full sit-ups or planks.
 - Focus on engaging the deep core muscles, including the transverse abdominis, through gentle abdominal contractions and breathing exercises.
 - Gradually progress to exercises that promote proper alignment and healing of the abdominal muscles, under the guidance of a qualified instructor.

3. Pelvic Floor Dysfunction:

- Modify exercises that put excessive pressure on the pelvic floor, such as deep squats or heavy lifting.

- Emphasize pelvic floor awareness and gentle exercises to strengthen and release the muscles, such as pelvic floor contractions (Kegels).

- Avoid exercises that cause straining or bearing down, and focus on maintaining good alignment and breathing techniques.

4. Low Back Pain:

- Modify exercises that exacerbate low back pain, such as deep forward folds or intense backbends.

- Focus on exercises that promote core stability and strengthen the deep abdominal and back muscles, such as pelvic tilts and gentle back extensions.

- Incorporate exercises that improve flexibility and mobility in the hips, hamstrings, and thoracic spine.

5. Shoulder or Neck Injuries:

- Modify exercises that put strain on the shoulders or neck, such as overhead movements or high planks.

- Use props or modifications to support the upper body and reduce strain, such as performing exercises with the hands on a higher surface or using lighter resistance.

- Focus on exercises that improve stability and mobility in the scapulae and upper back, while avoiding excessive strain on the injured area.

6. Joint Issues (e.g., arthritis, osteoporosis):

- Avoid high-impact exercises or movements that exacerbate joint pain or discomfort.

- Modify exercises to reduce joint stress, such as using a smaller range of motion or performing exercises in a seated or supported position.

- Focus on gentle strengthening exercises that promote joint stability and flexibility, and consult with your healthcare provider for specific guidelines.

Always consult with a qualified healthcare professional or a certified Pilates instructor who can assess your individual condition or injury and provide appropriate modifications. They can guide you in selecting exercises that are safe and beneficial for your specific needs, ensuring a positive and effective Pilates practice.

CELEBRATING YOUR POST-PREGNANCY PILATES JOURNEY

Celebrating your post-pregnancy Pilates journey is a wonderful way to acknowledge your progress, achievements, and the dedication you've put into your fitness and well-being. Here are some ideas for celebrating your journey:

1. Reflect on your achievements: Take a moment to reflect on how far you've come since starting your post-pregnancy Pilates journey. Consider the improvements in your strength, flexibility, posture, and

overall well-being. Celebrate the small milestones and the progress you've made along the way.

2. Set new goals: As you celebrate your achievements, set new goals to continue your post-pregnancy Pilates journey. Perhaps you want to master a challenging exercise, increase your flexibility, or incorporate new Pilates equipment into your practice. Setting goals will help you stay motivated and continue progressing.

3. Share your journey: Share your post-pregnancy Pilates journey with others. Talk to your friends, family, or other postpartum individuals who may be interested in starting a fitness routine. Share your experiences, the benefits you've gained, and how

Pilates has positively impacted your post-pregnancy recovery. Your journey may inspire and motivate others to embark on their own fitness journeys.

4. Treat yourself: Treat yourself to something special as a reward for your dedication and hard work. It could be a massage, a new workout outfit, a day of relaxation, or any other indulgence that makes you feel good. Celebrating your journey with a well-deserved treat can be a great way to pamper yourself and acknowledge your efforts.

5. Take progress photos: Document your progress by taking before-and-after photos or progress photos along the way. It can be incredibly motivating and satisfying to see the physical changes and

improvements in your body. You can keep these photos for yourself or share them with others to inspire and encourage their own fitness journeys.

6. Join a community: Connect with other postpartum individuals or individuals who share a passion for Pilates. Join a postnatal Pilates group, participate in online forums or social media communities, or find a workout buddy who can join you in your Pilates sessions. Building connections with like-minded individuals can provide support, accountability, and a sense of camaraderie as you celebrate your post-pregnancy Pilates journey together.

Remember, celebrating your post-pregnancy Pilates journey is not just about the destination but also about recognizing and appreciating the effort, commitment, and growth you've experienced along the way. Embrace the joy of your achievements and continue to prioritize your well-being as you move forward in your fitness journey.

Maintaining a Sustainable Exercise Routine

Maintaining a sustainable exercise routine is essential for long-term health and well-being. Here are some tips to help you establish and sustain a routine that works for you:

1. Set realistic goals: Start by setting realistic and achievable goals for your exercise routine. Consider your

current fitness level, time constraints, and other commitments. Setting small, attainable goals will help you stay motivated and build momentum.

2. Find activities you enjoy: Choose exercises and activities that you genuinely enjoy. Whether it's Pilates, yoga, swimming, dancing, or hiking, selecting activities you find fun and engaging increases the likelihood of sticking with them in the long run.

3. Prioritize consistency over intensity: Consistency is key when it comes to maintaining an exercise routine. Aim for regular workouts, even if they're shorter or less intense. It's better to have consistent, shorter workouts than sporadic, intense sessions. Consistency

builds habits and allows for gradual progress.

4. Schedule your workouts: Treat your exercise routine as an important appointment by scheduling it into your calendar. Set specific times and days for your workouts, making it a regular part of your routine. Treat it as a non-negotiable commitment to yourself.

5. Make it convenient: Choose exercise options that are convenient for your lifestyle. It could mean finding a Pilates studio or gym close to your home or workplace, setting up a home workout space, or incorporating physical activity into your daily routine, such as walking or cycling for transportation.

6. Be flexible and adaptable: Life can be unpredictable, and there may be times when your routine needs to be adjusted. Rather than getting discouraged, embrace flexibility and be open to modifying your exercise plans when necessary. Adapt to changes in your schedule or circumstances without giving up on your overall commitment to regular physical activity.

7. Set realistic time expectations: Recognize that there may be periods when you have more time and energy for longer workouts and other times when shorter workouts are more realistic. Be flexible with the duration and intensity of your workouts,

adapting them to fit your current circumstances.

8. Find an accountability system: Accountability can help you stay on track with your exercise routine. Find an accountability partner, join a fitness group or class, or use fitness apps or trackers to monitor your progress. Having someone or something to hold you accountable can provide motivation and support.

9. Listen to your body: Pay attention to your body's cues and adjust your routine accordingly. Rest when you need it, modify exercises if you're feeling fatigued or recovering from an injury, and seek professional guidance if necessary. Taking care of your body

and avoiding burnout is crucial for long-term sustainability.

10. Celebrate milestones and progress: Celebrate your achievements along the way. Acknowledge and reward yourself for reaching milestones, achieving personal bests, or consistently maintaining your exercise routine. Celebrating your progress can boost motivation and reinforce positive habits.

Remember, a sustainable exercise routine is not about perfection or adhering to a rigid plan. It's about finding a balance that works for you, enjoying the process, and making physical activity a lifelong habit that supports your overall well-being.

www.ingramcontent.com/pod-product-compliance
Lightning Source LLC
Chambersburg PA
CBHW070935260726
48661CB00003B/1002